SAQs in Clinical Surgery-in-General for the FRCS

SAQs in Clinical Surgery-in-General for the FRCS

Mr K.M. Mokbel
MB, BS(London), FRCS(England)
Department of General Surgery, The Chelsea and Westminster Hospital, Fulham Road, London SW10, UK

with a Foreword by
Robert Ham
Consultant Vascular and General Surgeon, The Royal London Hospital, London, UK

PETROC PRESS

Petroc Press, an imprint of LibraPharm Limited

Distributors

Plymbridge Distributors Limited, Plymbridge House, Estover Road, Plymouth PL6 7PZ, UK

Published in the United Kingdom by LibraPharm Limited, *Gemini House*, 162 Craven Road, Newbury, Berkshire RG14 5NR, UK

A catalogue record for this book is available from the British Library

ISBN 1 900603 90 X

Printed and bound in the United Kingdom by Hartnolls Limited, Bodmin, Cornwall

Contents

SAQs

PAPER I

PAPER II

PAPER III

PAPER IV

PAPER V

Foreword

The second part of the FRCS examination represents a testing and stressful, but, one hopes, ultimately rewarding experience. Preparation for all examinations should include not only study and revision but also practice in the techniques required to make optimal use of the knowledge acquired.

This volume provides an opportunity to practise the written part of the examination, but could also be used, with the help of a colleague, to practise viva technique. It will not only enable the acquisition of knowledge and its presentation to be tested, and new information added, but should ideally provide reassurance that progress is being made.

A wealth of practice questions and answers are provided. It is not anticipated that all the answers are complete, and it should be remembered that some questions are more relevant than others. Not all the information in this book is required by everyone who will pass the examination, but the methodology and principles of presentation will be familiar to many who do.

Good Luck!

Robert Ham
Consultant Vascular and General Surgeon
The Royal London Hospital

September 1993

Introduction

The book contains 40 surgical topics relevant to general surgical training in the form of short answer questions (SAQs) and short notes. Although it is primarily aimed at candidates preparing for the Clinical Surgery in General Section of the FRCS examination, it should be useful to all surgeons in training (junior and senior).

The stimulus for writing this book came from the major changes to the FRCS examination which took place in September 1990 (England). The written section of the new FRCS Part II examination consists of eight short answer questions (SAQs) and one long essay. This book provides a wealth of practice of SAQs with answers provided in the form of short notes, the form required in the examination and with which the candidate should become familiar. The answers in this book represent concise up-dated accounts of 40 topics thought to be important to general surgical training and relevant to the new syllabus guide published by the Royal College of Surgeons. Topics like trauma, organ transplantation, surgical audit, AIDS, the management of the burned patient and medical imaging have been covered. It should be remembered that this book is not meant to be comprehensive but to provide a revision guide for candidates preparing for the FRCS Part II examination. It will be useful to other surgeons in training and the senior undergraduate.

K.M. Mokbel
September 1993, London

FRCS PART II:
Tips on passing the examination

I. The written paper

In England, the written examination in clinical surgery in general consists of one paper lasting 3 hours and comprising:

A. A 2-hour short answer paper where you are asked to write short notes on eight selected topics (15 minutes per topic). Your notes should be as concise as possible.

B. A 1-hour essay.

When answering the written paper remember to:

1. Write clearly and legibly.
2. Use correct English and good grammar.
3. Use numbered underlined headings (in block capitals).
4. Reduce underlining to a minimum.
5. Adopt a well-spaced lay-out; this allows you to correct mistakes without causing much untidiness.
6. Use illustrations when necessary.
7. Be as concise as possible.

When answering short answer questions:

8. Attempt answering all questions satisfactorily as it is extremely difficult to recover from a poorly-answered or unanswered question because of the close marking system.
9. Avoid using abbreviations, e.g. CVP, IVP.
10. Do not be too controversial in your answer.
11. Follow the format when answering essay questions:
    a) Introduction (opening paragraph).
    b) Main body.
    c) Conclusion (closing paragraph).
12. Review your answers before leaving the examination room.

II. The vivas

There are two 20-minute vivas (Eng.); one on operative surgery and the other on various surgical topics, e.g. post-operative complications.

1. Dress smartly but conservatively, avoid casual jackets, loud suits, loud ties, short skirts, etc.
2. Make sure that your hair is not too long and you are clean shaven.
3. Appear confident and look the examiner in the eye.
4. Use concise, clear and simple English, in an audible voice.
5. Do not antagonize the examiners!
6. In the operative viva when you are asked to describe an operation try to use the following methodical system (unless you are asked by the examiner to omit certain steps):
   a) Pre-operative preparation, e.g. informed consent; heparinization for femoral embolectomy; bowel preparation for bowel surgery; premedication.
   b) Anaesthetic, local or general.
   c) Positioning the patient on the table.
   d) Skin cleansing and drapes.
   e) Incision.
   f) Initial assessment of findings.
   g) Procedure (including recognized difficulties and hazards).
   h) Closure.
   i) Drains (if required).
   j) Post-operative care (including treatment, investigations, and nursing care).

III. The clinicals

Dress smartly but conservatively.

A. The long case.
   - Plan and allocate your time carefully.
   - Establish a good rapport with the patient.
   - Be thorough in your history taking and physical examination.
   - Always plan to have time at the end of the long case to prepare your presentation, think about the diagnosis, investigations and any points the examiners might raise in the discussion.

- Make your presentation as concise and interesting as possible. Start by stating the patient's name and age.
- Avoid mentioning many negative findings.
- Avoid using abbreviations, e.g. JVP.

B. The short cases.
- The best method of preparing for the short cases is to examine patients repeatedly in front of an observer.
- Always introduce yourself to the patients, shake hands with them and get their permission to examine them.
- Follow the examiner's instructions carefully.
- Position the patient correctly and get an adequate exposure of the part to be examined.
- Follow the correct steps of the examination (starting with observation) and move on smoothly from one step to the other. After presenting your positive findings (in a methodical sequence) state the diagnosis or a possible diagnosis and give differential diagnosis. For example when examining a lump (e.g. lipoma) follow the following sequence: 1) position; 2) colour; 3) tenderness; 4) local temperature; 5) shape; 6) size; 7) surface; 8) edge; 9) composition; 10) relations; and 11) regional lymph nodes.
- The examiner may ask you for a running commentary as you are performing the examination.
- Avoid using words such as 'I think', 'it might be', 'I'm not sure', etc.
- Always thank the patients at the end and help them to dress.

Good Luck!

PAPER I

QUESTIONS

Write short notes on:

1. The compartment syndrome.
2. Malignant skin melanoma.
3. Tracheostomy.
4. Complications of ulcerative colitis.
5. The clinical applications of ultrasound in urology.
6. The flail chest.
7. The clinical presentation, diagnosis and treatment of thyroid cancer
8. Extradural haematoma.

ANSWERS

1. The compartment syndrome

- Nerves can survive ischaemia for 2–4 hours but can potentially regenerate.
- Muscle can survive 6–8 hours, but infarction is irreversible leading to fibrotic contractures (Volkmann's ischaemic contractures).
- The forearm compartments (anterior and posterior) and the lower leg compartments (anterior tibial, peroneal and deep posterior) are the commonest sites.
- Common causes include fractures of the elbow (especially supracondylar fractures), forearm and proximal tibia.

Signs and symptoms
- The 5 P's may be present in the hands or feet, e.g. paralysis, pallor or cyanosis, paraesthesiae, pain and pulselessness (may be a late feature).
- Tightness and tenderness in the forearm or calf.

- Pain (in the forearm flexors or the lower leg muscles) when passively extending the fingers or the foot. This pain may be agonizing and may be in excess of that expected from the injury sustained.

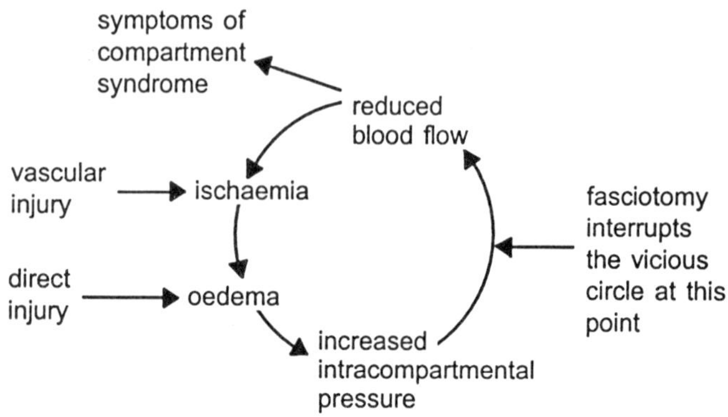

Figure. The vicious circle of compartment syndrome

Investigations
- Plain radiographs to show the fracture (if any).
- Measurement of intracompartmental pressure using a cannula and a transducer.
- A pressure >30 mmHg indicates urgent action.

Treatment
- The syndrome should be diagnosed without delay before extensive irreversible damage has occurred.
- If an artery is thought to be kinked by a fracture, an immediate reduction is performed.
- In the threatened syndrome an extensive fasciotomy is performed, the arteries are explored and dealt with appropriately (ligation, excision, grafting, etc.), the wound is left open for 5 days then inspected. If there is necrotic muscle, debridement is carried out and the wound is closed without tension.
- The limb should be cooled down to lower its metabolic rate.
- Long-term physiotherapy may help in reducing the severity of the contractures.

2. Malignant skin melanoma

Aetiology

- Exposure of white skin to solar radiation.
- About 40% arise in a pre-existing mole (change in colour, size, elevation and outline, itching, bleeding or tingling should raise suspicion).
- Familial clustering (especially with dysplastic naevus).
- Immunosuppression.

Clinical types

1. Lentigo maligna – 7% of cases. Least malignant.
2. Superficial spreading – 65% of cases. Horizontal growth phase.
3. Nodular. Most malignant. Vertical growth phase.
4. Amelanotic (rare).
5. Acral lentiginous (hands and feet) is as malignant as nodular.

Pathological classification

A. Clark's levels from I (intra-epidermal) to V (invasion of subcutaneous tissue).
B. Breslow thickness in mm using optical micrometer.

Clinical staging

Stage I: Cutaneous melanoma only.
Stage IIa: As in I plus satellite or in-transit deposits.
Stage IIb: Regional lymphadenopathy is present.
Stage III: Distant metastases are present.

Investigation

- Excision biopsy (histology Clark's level and Breslow thickness defined).
- CXR, LFTs, bone profile, US/CT staging, and bone scan may be required.

Factors influencing prognosis

1. Clark's level and Breslow thickness.
2. Clinical stage.
3. Site of tumour (worse prognosis for head and trunk than for extremities).
4. Sex (females have better prognosis).

5. Age (younger patients have better prognosis).

Treatment

Stage I: Surgical excision of primary tumour using a no-touch technique and including a clear margin (0.5–2.0 cm). The dimensions of excision depend upon thickness of tumour and anatomical site. Plastic reconstruction with skin grafts or flaps may be necessary.

Stage IIa: Surgical excision of primary tumour.
- If melanoma thicker than 1 mm then prophylactic lymph node dissection may be carried out.
- Lasers, cryotherapy, electron radiotherapy and isolated limb perfusion have been used.

Stage IIb: Surgical excision and block dissection of regional lymph nodes.

Stage III: There is no established treatment for this stage.
- Prognosis is very poor in advanced melanoma.
- Dacarbazime, vindesine, IL-2 and/or interferons are relatively effective agents. Tumour necrosis factor and BCG have also been used.
- Surgery has a role in the local control of extensive skin disease.

3. Tracheostomy

Indications

1. Upper airway obstruction.
   a) Congenital e.g. subglottic stenosis, laryngeal web, laryngeal cysts, laryngeal haemangioma, etc.
   b) Trauma e.g. prolonged endotracheal intubation, penetrating injuries, steam inhalation, etc.
   c) Tumours e.g. advanced carcinoma of the tongue, larynx and trachea, carcinoma of thyroid.
   d) Infections e.g. acute epiglottitis, laryngo-tracheo-bronchitis, diphtheria.
   e) Foreign body.
   f) Bilateral abductor paralysis of vocal cords.
   g) Post-thyroidectomy haemorrhage.

2. Respiratory failure due to pulmonary disease, structural abnormalities of the thoracic cage or neuromuscular dysfunction.

3. Protection of the tracheo-bronchial tree in conditions such as coma, brain stem infarction, myasthenia gravis, Guillain-Barré syndrome, tetanus and multiple facial injuries.

Urgent or elective

- In life-threatening upper airway obstruction, laryngotomy (opening the cricothyroid membrane) is preferred to urgent tracheostomy.
- In elective tracheostomy (GA, endotracheal intubation) a transverse incision is made midway between the cricoid cartilage and suprasternal notch. The straps are retracted and the thyroid isthmus is divided. An elliptical disc is cut out centred on the 3rd and 4th tracheal ring, then a tube is inserted. The cut thyroid ends are usually sutured.

Tracheostomy tubes

Various types are available.

1. Negus tube (upper airway obstruction).
2. Cuffed plastic tube (airway protection and positive pressure ventilation).
3. Alder Hey tube (infants and children).

Complications

1. Dislodgement of the tube (partial or complete).
2. Obstruction of the tube or trachea by crusts of secretion.
3. Surgical emphysema.
4. Subglottic stenosis if 1st or 2nd tracheal rings are damaged.
5. Pneumothorax if pleural dome is damaged.
6. Pulmonary infection is the most frequent complication.
7. Late tracheal stenosis (tracheal ischaemia due to a cuffed tube).
8. Air embolism.
9. Sepsis.
10. Cuff prolapse causing obstruction.
11. Intubation granuloma of vocal cords.
12. Haemorrhage which may be fatal.

---

4. Complications of ulcerative colitis

1. Acute toxic dilatation.
   - Occurs in about 6–13% of patients.
   - Plain abdominal X-rays show a thick-walled dilated colon with luminal gas and mucosal islands.
   - If patient does not improve within 48 hours on high-dose corticosteroids, emergency surgery may become necessary. Medical treatment is attempted in the first 48 hours provided the condition is stable otherwise immediate surgery is indicated.

2. Perforation of the colon.
   - Occurs in about 4% of hospitalized patients (may be as high as 19% in severe total involvement).
   - Commonest in the sigmoid colon or splenic flexure.
   - May result in a localized abscess or generalized peritonitis.

3. Haemorrhage. It is rarely massive. About half the cases occur in association with toxic megacolon.

4. Stricture. Occurs in about 10% of cases.

5. Colorectal carcinoma.
   - Incidence is about 20% after 20 years of disease.
   - Regular sigmoidoscopy and colonoscopy with multiple biopsies are required.
   - Prophylactic restorative proctocolectomy should be considered.

6. Anal fissures occur in about 10% of cases.

7. Anal fistulas.

8. Ano-rectal abscesses.

9. Extra-gastrointestinal manifestations.
   a) Eye complications occur in about 4% of cases (uveitis, episcleritis and conjunctivitis).
   b) Arthropathy (monoarticular arthritis and ankylosing spondylitis) occurs in 10% of cases.

c) Skin (erythema nodosum, erythema multiforme, pyoderma gangrenosum and aphthous stomatitis).
d) Hepatobiliary manifestations include fatty change (common), pericholangitis (25% of cases), sclerosing cholangitis (10% of cases), chronic active hepatitis, cirrhosis and possibly carcinoma of the bile duct and pancreatic insufficiency.
e) Malnutrition.
f) Iron deficiency anaemia.

10. Complications of therapy.
    - Anti-inflammatory drugs.
    - Immunosuppressants.
    - Surgery.

---

5. The clinical applications of ultrasound in urology

Advantages: non-invasive, no radiation, no contrast media, inexpensive, portable and imaging is possible in many planes.

Diagnostic uses

1. Kidney and ureter.
   The echogenicity of the normal kidney is increased in the pelvicalyceal sinus fat complex, decreased in the pyramids and intermediate in the cortex.
   a) Congenital disorders. Ultrasound (US) is valuable in the diagnosis of aplastic or hypoplastic kidneys (compensatory hypertrophy of contralateral kidney), horseshoe kidney and polycystic kidneys (enlarged with numerous cysts).
   b) Renal masses. Lesions >1 cm are easily detected by US. Uncomplicated cysts appear as well-delineated circular lesions lacking internal echoes. Solid tumours show mixed echogenicity. US cannot distinguish between malignant and benign tumours (angiomyolipoma is an exception). US is valuable in staging malignant tumours (liver deposits, lymphadenopathy) and in the follow-up of nephrectomy. US-guided needle aspiration of lesions is useful diagnostically.
   c) Inflammation. In acute pyelonephritis the kidney is grossly enlarged. The enlargement is focal in the focal form. In chronic atrophic pyelonephritis the kidney is small with focal increase in echogenicity due to fibrosis. An abscess appears to have an irregular thick wall and low-amplitude central echoes.
   d) Calcification presents as increased echogenicity which is sharply defined.
   e) Hydronephrosis. There is splaying of the pelvicalyceal sinus fat echo complex. A cause of obstruction may be identified by US.
   f) Renal transplantation. US is valuable in the diagnosis of acute rejection (enlarged kidney with prominent pyramids) and pararenal collections.
   g) US is useful in the initial assessment of renal injuries following abdominal trauma.

2. Bladder and prostate.
   - Transabdominal US (with a urine-filled bladder) can detect bladder diverticula, calculi and tumours. Tumour staging is not sensitive.
   - Transrectal US is useful in measuring residual urine, size and weight of prostate. BPH presents a sharply delineated capsule whereas prostatic carcinoma show disruption of the capsule with asymmetry. US-guided needle biopsy of prostate is possible.
   - Transrectal/transurethral US may allow accurate staging of bladder tumour.

3. Scrotum.
   - Malignant testicular tumours are usually echo-poor.
   - Occult testicular tumours can be identified.
   - Hydrocele presents as an echo-free area surrounding the testis.
   - Epididymal cysts and spermatoceles have the US appearance of a cyst.
   - US cannot distinguish torsion from epididymo-orchitis.
   - US is useful in evaluating testicular trauma and undescended testes.

Therapeutic uses

US scanning allows the following percutaneous procedures to be performed.

1. Catheter drainage of an abscess.
2. Nephrostomy catheter drainage of an obstructed kidney.
3. Endopyeloplasty.
4. Perfusion chemolysis of renal calculi.
5. Percutaneous nephrolithotomy for renal calculi.
6. Percutaneous resection and coagulation of urothelial tumours.

Calculi can be fragmented by ultrasonic nephrolithotripsy.

---

6. The flail chest

Pathology

- Occurs in about 20% of significant blunt thoracic trauma.
- One portion of the chest wall becomes isolated due to multiple fractures (usually two fractures of the same rib), costochondral separation or detachment from the transverse process of the vertebral body.
- Respiratory failure results from pulmonary contusion, paradoxical chest movement (↑ dead space, mediastinal shift) and pain.

Principles of management

1. Immediate treatment of mechanical problems, e.g. airway obstruction, haemopneumothorax.
2. Early stabilization by local support.
3. Crystalloid infusion is limited to 1 litre during initial resuscitation, plasma protein fraction, colloids and blood are used to restore circulatory volume. Diuretics may be used.
4. If $PaO_2 > 8$ kPa, $PaCO_2 < 8$ kPa, RR < 35/min and FVC > 15 ml/kg, the patient can be managed conservatively without mechanical ventilation.
5. CPAP with or without IMV is used if
   - $PaO_2 < 8$ kPa, $PaCO_2 > 8$ kPa, RR > 35/min and FVC < 15 ml/kg.
   - Patient is severely shocked.
   - General anaesthesia is required.
   - Pre-existing lung disease is present.

   The patient is kept on the ITU for 2–5 days and returned to the wards if pain is well controlled and cough is effective.
6. Pain control with epidural anaesthesia, intercostal nerve block, i.m. opiate or oral codeine.
7. Chest physiotherapy coinciding with periods of maximum pain relief.
8. Sputum is sent for culture and infections are treated with the appropriate antimicrobials.

7. The clinical presentation, diagnosis and treatment of thyroid cancer

Clinical presentation

- Rapid and progressive growth of single or dominant thyroid nodules which may be fixed to underlying structures.
- Enlarged lymph nodes in the neck.
- Diffuse thyroid enlargement (anaplastic or lymphoma).
- Recurrent laryngeal nerve palsy (hoarse voice).
- Dysphagia or respiratory obstruction.

Investigation

- Thyroid function tests to rule out thyrotoxicosis.
- Serum calcitonin, if medullary carcinoma is suspected.
- Ultrasound has significant limitations in identifying malignant disease.
- Isotope scanning. Malignant disease is found in approximately 15% of cold nodules and in 10% of warm nodules. This investigation also has limitations.
- Fine-needle aspiration biopsy is a simple, safe and effective technique in assessing the probability of malignancy in thyroid nodules. It requires cytological expertise. In expert hands false negative and false positive rates are low.
- It is impossible to differentiate on a cytological basis between benign follicular adenoma and a follicular carcinoma.
- Frozen section at operation is preoperative diagnosis is not established.

Management

1. Well-differentiated thyroid cancer is treated initially with a total thyroidectomy and removal of involved lymph nodes. Aggressive neck dissection does not seem to improve survival.

2. Medullary cancer is treated with a total thyroidectomy plus central node dissection.

3. Anaplastic carcinoma is treated palliatively with local removal, chemotherapy and/or radiotherapy. The prognosis is poor.

4. Lymphoma. Chemotherapy and radiotherapy are the main treatment nodalities. Surgery is required either to establish the diagnosis or relieve tracheal compression.

5. Replacement therapy with thyroxine is required in total thyroidectomy patients.

6. Following total thyroidectomy, ablative dose of radioactive iodine ^{131}I is administered. Serum thyroglobulin levels and follow-up radioactive iodine scans are used to detect recurrence. Complications of total thyroidectomy include recurrent laryngeal nerve palsy (which may be bilateral), haemorrhage, external laryngeal nerve palsy and hypoparathyroidsim. Radioactive iodine administration increases the incidence of leukaemia and lymphoma.

---

8. Extradural haematoma

- Source of bleeding may be arterial (middle meningeal artery) or venous (sagittal and transverse sinuses).
- Is associated with a skull fracture in about 95% of adults (lower percentage in children who have pliant skulls).
- Initially the brain compensates for the haematoma (lucid interval).
- There may be a history of head injury followed by concussion with relatively rapid recovery followed by the lucent interval and then deterioration.

Symptoms and signs

1. Increased intracranial pressure (ICP).
   a) Headaches.
   b) Vomiting and nausea.
   c) Neck stiffness.
   d) Papilloedema.
   e) 3rd nerve palsy (pupillary dilatation) due to tentorial herniation.
   f) Impairment of consciousness.
   g) False localizing signs.

2. Focal brain damage.
   a) Hemiplegia or hemianaesthesia (contralateral).
   b) Dysphasia if dominant hemisphere is affected.
   c) Homonomous hemianopia due to damage to the occipital and parietal lobes.
   d) Ataxia, diplopia and nystagmus in posterior cranial haematoma.
   e) Seizures.

   Note: Contralateral hemiparesis is an early sign whereas ipsilateral hemiparesis is a late sign.

3. There may be boggy swelling beneath the temporalis muscle.

Investigations

1. Plain radiographs of the skull, cervical spine and chest. A skull fracture is seen in about 95% of cases in adults.

2. CT scan is indicated if there are
   a) Focal signs.

b) Fluctuating or deteriorating level of consciousness.
c) Epileptic seizure.
d) Penetrating head injury.
e) Combination of head and facial injuries.

3. Arterial blood gases.

4. FBC, plasma urea and electrolytes (U + E) and group and save (G + S).

Management

1. Secure an adequate airway and effective breathing – the indications for controlled ventilation include an associated chest injury, emergency reduction of ICP, aspiration pneumonia, control of epilepsy and diffuse cerebral oedema.
2. Assessment (primary and secondary survey) – the assessment includes a Glasgow Coma Score (GCS).
3. Fluid replacement should be carefully controlled – severe closed head injuries require little fluid replacement. Urinary catheterization may be necessary.
4. Early administration of mannitol and dexamethasone in order to reduce ICP.
5. Analgesia.
6. Half-hourly neuro-observation.
7. Surgery – should not be delayed by investigations. If the patient is deteriorating rapidly an emergency burr hole should be performed to evacuate the haematoma guided by the site of the fracture and the side of pupillary dilatation. Frontal, parietal and temporal holes may be performed; if all are negative on one side, burr holes should be repeated on the other side. Nowadays CT scanning determines the site of the craniotomy (craniotomy should be preferably performed by the neurosurgeon). Other surgical procedures such as elevation of depressed skull fractures and craniectomy may be required.

   Note: If the ipsilateral pupil is dilated, the dura should be opened to explore for and relieve possible hippocampal herniation. If the site of the bleeding is not obvious, pack the foramen spinosum with wax.

PAPER II

QUESTIONS

Write short notes on:

1. The principles of management of compound fractures.
2. Intussusception.
3. Treatment of thyrotoxicosis.
4. Diagnosis and management of pancreatic carcinoma.
5. Renal injuries.
6. Lasers in gastrointestinal surgery.
7. Adult respiratory distress syndrome.
8. The pre-operative management of the jaundiced patient.

ANSWERS

1. The principles of management of compound fractures

Classification

Type I
- Clean skin laceration <1 cm.
- No crush injury.
- Minimal soft tissue damage.
- Simple fracture (non-comminuted).

Type II
- Skin laceration >2 cm.
- Extensive soft tissue damage.
- Minimal to moderate crush injury.
- Simple fracture.

Type III
- High energy injury.
- Significant crush injury.
- Severe soft tissue damage.
- Comminuted fracture.

Principles of treatment

1. Compound fractures are surgical emergencies and should be treated within 6 hours of injury.
2. Wound swabs are taken immediately, then the wound is covered with a sterile dressing soaked in antiseptic solution.
3. Broad-spectrum intravenous antibiotics (e.g. cefuroxime) are commenced in the accident and emergency department. Antibiotics should be continued for 3 days.
4. The patient is taken to theatre and the wound is formally explored. It is initially mechanically cleaned and washed with an antiseptic solution (e.g. cetrimide), then thoroughly irrigated with a few litres of normal saline. Any devitalized tissue is excised and formal fasciotomies are performed if compartment syndrome is suspected. Damage to blood vessels is dealt with accordingly. The ends of severed nerves may be lightly sutured, then repaired in a later operation.
5. Stabilization of the fracture. Skeletal traction and plaster cast are reserved for type I fractures, as excessive movement at the fracture site predisposes to infection. Type II and III fractures should be treated with rigid external or internal fixation. External fixation is widely used for type III fractures and is the treatment of choice for such fractures in the tibia and the pelvis. However, recent studies suggest that primary internal fixation may have a role in the management of type III fractures.
6. Wound closure. The wound can be primarily closed in type I fracture (avoid suturing under tension). Wounds of type II and III fractures are left open and dressed with a sterile covering, then reinspected 3 days later. If infection has been aborted a delayed primary closure is performed. However if infection is present, the wound is dressed daily with a sterile dry-to-moist dressing and allowed to heal by secondary intention. Skin grafting may be necessary.

2. Intussusception

Pathology

- Invagination of segment of bowel (intussusceptum) into the adjacent segment (intussuscipiens) (see Figure).

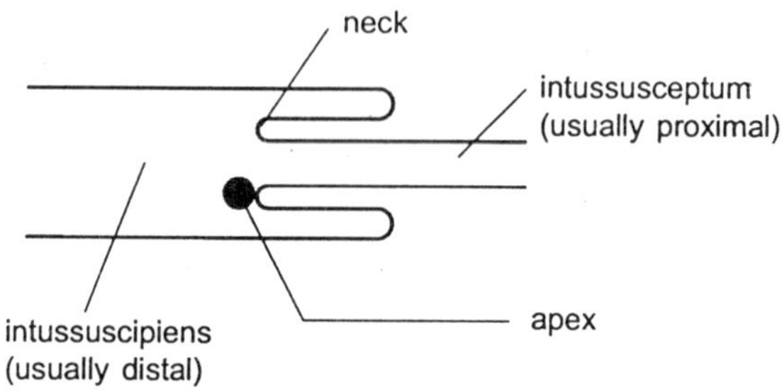

- Ileo-colic 77%, ileo-ileo-colic 12%, ileo-ileal 5%, colo-colic 2%.
- Commonest cause of bowel obstruction in children under 2.
- Peak age is about 7 months with M:F = 3:1.
- Most paediatric cases have no obvious cause, but there is a seasonal incidence and positive correlation with adenovirus infection and hypertrophic Peyer's patches.
- Other causes include: polyps, papilliferous carcinoma, submucous lipoma, intraluminal haematoma, inverted Meckel's diverticulum and intestinal lymphoma.
- The process may result in gangrene and perforation.

Symptoms

- Intermittent abdominal colic associated with crying and pallor followed by a period of wellbeing.
- Abdominal distension, vomiting, fever, lethargy, currant jelly stools and eventually shock.

Signs

- Abdominal distension.
- Dance's sign (empty right iliac fossa (RIF) and sausage-like mass in the right upper quadrant (RUQ)/epigastrium) (see Figure overleaf).

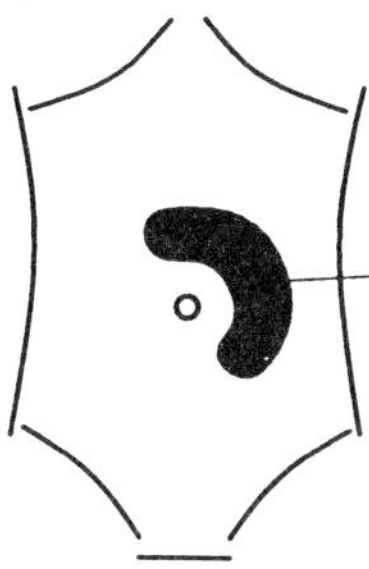

Investigations
- FBC (↑white cell count, haemoconcentration).
- Plasma U + E's and creatinine (dehydration).
- Barium enema usually confirms the diagnosis ('claw' sign may be seen in the ileo-colic type).
- Isotope abdominal scan may outline the intussusception.
- Signs of peritonitis and shock.

Treatment
- Correction of hypovolaemia and dehydration.
- Reduction by hydrostatic pressure using normal saline or barium reservoir connected to a lubricated catheter passed per rectum. Fluoroscopic imaging is required.
- If hydrostatic reduction is unsuccessful or equivocal, operative reduction is resorted to through a right lower quadrant transverse incision. Reduction is achieved through gentle retrograde compression (never pull).
- Irreducible or gangrenous intussusception is resected.
- Mikulicz procedure may be used in critically ill patients.

Prognosis
Recurrence rates 3% in enema reductions and 1.5% in operative reductions.

3. Treatment of thyrotoxicosis

1. Antithyroid drugs.

a) Carbimazole (the drug of choice).

   - Its metabolite methimazole acts as a substrate for peroxidase thus diverting oxidized iodine from incorporation into thyroglobulin. It also reduces iodination of tyrosine and coupling of iodotyrosines.
   - Indicated in patients under 18, pregnant women and small toxic goitre.
   - 10–15 mg tds initially. Maintenance dose is 10–20 mg daily.
   - Patient becomes euthyroid in about 3 months. Maintenance is continued for 1–2 years.
   - Side-effects include hair loss, skin rashes, agranulocytosis, drug fever and arthralgia.
   - Maintenance thyroxine may be required.
   - Relapse rate is about 70% at 5 years.

b) Propylthiouracil is similar to carbimazole.

c) Potassium perchlorate.

2. β-Blockers, e.g. propanolol.

- Control symptoms such as tachycardia, anxiety and tremor. They also block conversion of T3 and T4 in tissues.
- May be used in conjunction with anti-thyroid drugs, in thyrotoxic crisis and pre-operatively before subtotal thyroidectomy for thyrotoxicosis.

3. Sub-total thyroidectomy.

- Indications:
  a) Failure of medical treatment.
  b) Large toxic goitre.
  c) Patient preference for surgery.
  d) Exclusion of malignancy.
  e) Poor compliance with medical treatment.
  f) Intolerance of side-effects of anti-thyroid drugs.
- Most of the thyroid tissue is removed.
- Lugol's iodine may be given for 10 days pre-operatively.
- Propranolol may be given pre-operatively.
- Complications:

a) Recurrent laryngeal nerve palsy.
   - Incidence is about 1%.
b) Hypoparathyroidism.
   - Incidence is about 1%.
   - Always check serum Ca^{2+} postoperatively.
c) Hypothyroidism.
   - Incidence is about 20%.
   - Thyroxine is required.
d) External laryngeal nerve palsy (1–5%).
e) Recurrent thyrotoxicosis.
f) Haemorrhage.

4. *Radio-active iodine (^{131}I).*
   - Chief problem is to calculate the right dose.
   - Avoid in children, young adults and pregnancy.
   - Rate of hypothyroidism is about 75% at 10 years (thyroid function tests should be performed at yearly intervals for at least 10 years).

5. *Thyrotoxic crisis.*
   - Hyperpyrexia, hyperkinesis, dehydration, cardiac failure, tachycardia and shock are the main clinical features.
   - Treatment includes β-blockers, antithyroid drugs, i.v. fluids, cooling, steroids, oxygen, digoxin, diuretic and potassium iodide.

6. *Ophthalmic complications.*
   - Severe cases require high dose steroids, azathioprine or surgical decompression of the orbit. Total thyroidectomy is not recommended.
   - Mild cases may be treated with 5% guanethidine eye drops, protective glasses and lateral tarsorrhaphy.

---

4. Diagnosis and management of pancreatic carcinoma

Clinical features

- Usually middle-aged or elderly patients.
- Upper abdominal pain (80%).
- Vague abdominal pain with negative endoscopies.
- Pain may radiate to back (30%).
- Obstructive jaundice (75% of cases); the jaundice may be painless.
- Unexplained diabetes mellitus (6%).
- Unexplained acute pancreatitis (4%).
- Significant weight loss.

Investigations

These are initiated in any middle-aged or elderly patient presenting with any of the features listed above.

1. FBC (low Hb in 60% of cases).
2. Biochemical profile (obstructive jaundice with raised alkaline phosphatase, ↑ blood glucose).
3. Abdominal ultrasound (US) by an experienced radiologist (sensitivity is about 95%). Endoscopic ultrasound is useful in localizing the tumour.
4. CT scanning: if US shows a mass or dilatation of the distal pancreatic duct with no liver secondaries then CT scan is performed.
5. ERCP for placement of an endoscopic stent (pre-operatively) and obtaining pancreatic secretions for cytology.
6. Selective visceral angiography to predict any vascular involvement may be performed prior to surgery in order to stage pancreatic cancer.

Management

- Resectable lesions include tumours confined to pancreas, tumours with soft tissue local invasion (no vascular involvement) and tumours with small local lymph nodes involved.
- For resectable tumours of the head a pancreaticoduodenectomy (Whipple's operation) is performed. If frozen sections of the neck show invasion then total pancreatectomy is performed. A pylorus preserving operation may be performed for small lesions of the head. Multicentric pancreatic tumours are effectively treated by total pancreatectomy.

- For unresectable lesions cholecystojejunostomy or choledochojejunostomy may be performed to relieve jaundice. Percutaneous or endoscopically placed stents may also be used for relief of jaundice.
- Adjuvant therapy includes a combination of radiotherapy and 5-fluorouracil.
- The use of tamoxifen as a treatment modality has been reported.
- Chemical or surgical destruction of the autonomic nerve supply to the pancreas (splanchnic) may relieve intractable pain.

Prognosis

5 year survival rate for tumours of the head of the pancreas is about 10%.

5. Renal injuries

Aetiology
Blunt trauma accounts for 85% of cases. Rapid deceleration is particularly associated with vascular injury. Penetrating wounds account for 15% of cases (a high incidence of associated abdominal visceral injuries – 80%).

History
History of trauma, pain (flank, abdomen, lower ribs), haematoma, and symptoms due to associated injuries.

Examinations
Signs of shock, bruising and tenderness (flank and abdomen), rib fractures, a palpable abdominal mass (haematoma or extravasated urine), signs of paralytic ileus.

Investigations:
1. Microscopy and dip testing of urine may reveal haematuria which may be absent in vascular injuries.
2. FBC, plasma, U + Es and creatinine.
3. Intravenous pyelogram (IVP) should outline the kidneys and collecting system and define the extent of injury. It should be performed in all patients who have macroscopic haematuria. If it fails to define the extent of injury a nephrotomogram may be performed.
4. Arteriography. The non-visualization of a kidney on an IVP can be due to two causes: (i) absent kidney (congenital or previous nephrectomy); (ii) vascular injuries (avulsion of the pedicle or renal artery thrombosis). In the latter situation an arteriogram is indicated.
5. CT scanning is excellent in assessing renal and associated abdominal injuries. The use of contrasts improves accuracy.
6. US is useful in the initial assessment.

Treatment
1. Emergency measures: initial resuscitation and treatment of shock if present.
2. Observations: the patient is nursed in bed and adequately hydrated. Pulse, BP and abdominal girth are regularly noted. Urine specimens

should be examined. Analgesics are prescribed as required. About 85% of cases settle with this conservative management.

3. Surgery: the indications for surgical exploration are:
   a) Signs of progressive haemorrhage.
   b) Significant extravasation of urine.
   c) Almost all penetrating injuries.
   d) Treatment of complications such as arteriovenous fistula, hydronephrosis, urinoma, perinephric abscess, etc.

Immediate exploration of renal injuries (when indicated) should be performed through a transperitoneal approach (midline incision) to allow control of renal vessels and assessment of damage to intraperitoneal contents. A delayed exploration may be performed through a loin incision. At exploration: renal lacerations are repaired; perinephric haematoma and extravasated urine are drained; partial or complete nephrectomy may be carried out; an attempt should be made to repair vascular injuries – however, if the renal pedicle is completely avulsed the kidney may be implanted in the contralateral iliac fossa.

Prognosis

Is excellent with proper management. Long-term follow-up to detect and treat complications (e.g. hypertension, hydronephrosis) is necessary.

---

6. Lasers in gastrointestinal surgery

Principles of lasers

The atoms in the laser medium are stimulated by a power source (optical or electrical) so that a population inversion is established. The excited atoms emit photons when the electrons move to a lower energy level (closer to the nucleus). This emission is amplified by multiple reflections between mirrors. Some of the emitted photons (with equal energy) escape through the partially reflecting mirror as the laser beam which is monochromatic. The interaction between the laser light and tissue depends on the wavelength of the light and the tissue composition. The extent and speed of the thermal injury is influenced by the laser medium. Laser light can be transmitted along quartz fibres.

Therapeutic applications

1. Bleeding peptic ulcer.
   - Thermal contraction of the feeding vessel by ringing the bleeding point by endoscopic laser.
   - Rebleeding rate is about 15%.

2. Angiodysplasia and haemorrhagic telangiectasia in the stomach, duodenum and colon (endoscopic).

3. Carcinoma of the oesophagus and gastric cardia.
   - Palliation of malignant dysphagia.
   - Indicated when tumour is incurable or the patient is unfit for surgery.
   - Especially suitable for high oesophageal lesions and anastomotic recurrence after oesophageal resection.

4. Inoperable rectosigmoid tumours.
   - Endoscopic NdYAG laser improves symptoms in 85% of cases.
   - Also suitable for anastomotic recurrence.

5. Colonic polyps.
   - Colonoscopic laser can be used to eradicate sessile and villous adenoma in the elderly with fewer complications than surgery.

6. Irradiation proctitis.

7. Haemorrhoidectomy.

8. Haemostasis of recurrent/inoperable gastric carcinoma.

9. CO_2 laser scalpel is used in liver resection minimizing bleeding.

Notes

A. Lasers are named according to the medium used. NdYAG laser is the one usually used in the procedures listed above.

B. Photodynamic therapy: A photosensitizing agent administered and selectively retained in the tumour is made to fluoresce when exposed to an appropriate laser light. This causes local cytotoxic damage in the presence of oxygen and may be useful in the treatment of small colorectal tumours (without reducing the mechanical strength of the bowel) and polyps in the upper GIT in familial polyposis coli.

Hazards

1. Accidental fires.
2. Eye damage; eyes (patient and surgeon) should be protected with safety glasses and reflective objects should be avoided.
3. Ignition of bowel gases.
4. Perforation of a viscus.

7. Adult respiratory distress syndrome (ARDS)

Pathology

- In the alveoli there is interstitial haemorrhage, oedema (protein-rich) and neutrophil infiltration.
- Depletion of type I pneumocytes.
- Functional disruption of the capillary-alveolar membrane.
- Fibrin deposition.
- Free radicals of oxygen, eicosanoids and endotoxin are thought to mediate the damage.
- About 10 aetiological factors have been identified – all impinging on lung ischaemia leading to thrombosis in situ or pulmonary emboli.

Clinical features

- Predisposing factors include sepsis, massive blood transfusions, multiple trauma, head injury, prolonged shock and pulmonary contusion.
- Usually presents 24–72 hours after injury.
- Dyspnoea, tachypnoea and tachycardia are the usual symptoms.
- PaO_2 < 10 kPa with FIO_2 > 0.5, pulmonary wedge pressure < 18 mmHg and widespread bilateral infiltrate on the chest X-ray are diagnostic.

Investigations

- Arterial blood gases ↓PaO_2, ↓PCO_2 (initially), ↑PCO_2 (later).
- Chest X-ray.
- CT scan of lungs allows quantification of lung damage and prediction of need for ventilation.
- Other tests ↓ lung compliance, ↓ FRC (functional residual capacity), ↑ perfusion/ventilation mismatch, ↑ right-to-left shunting.
- Normal pulmonary wedge pressure and lack of response to diuretics help to distinguish the condition from cardiac failure. It should be remembered, however, that heart failure may complicate ARDS in the later stages.

Treatment

1. Control of triggering factors, e.g. sepsis.
2. Correction of circulating volume.
3. Correction of hypoxaemia.
   a) In mild cases PaO_2 > 8 kPa humidified oxygen-enriched air is

given through venturi mask or nasal cannulae.

b) In severe cases PaO_2 < 8 kPa or lung damage >30% on CT scan ventilation is required. Two forms may be used: intermittent positive pressure ventilation (IPPV) or positive end expiratory pressure ventilation (PEEPV).

Note

Extracorporeal CO_2 removal with extracorporeal membrane oxygenator has been recently applied with success.

---

8. The pre-operative management of the jaundiced patient (obstructive jaundice)

1. Correction of fluid and electrolyte balance.
   - The main aim is to prevent post-operative renal failure.
   - There may be dilutional hyponatraemia.
   - Any hypokalaemia should be corrected.
   - 5% dextrose infusion is started 12 hours pre-operatively and i.v. mannitol or frusemide is started at induction. The patient is catheterized and the hourly urine output should be maintained above 35 ml/h peri- and post-operatively.

2. Correction of disordered haemostasis.
   - Vitamin K deficiency (obstructive jaundice) reduces the levels of vitamin K dependent factors. This can be corrected by giving vitamin K i.v. or i.m. 2–3 days pre-operatively.
   - In severe hepatic damage fresh frozen plasma is required.
   - Disseminated intravascular coagulopathy (DIC) may be present in jaundiced patients due to endotoxaemia and should be treated appropriately (e.g. FFP, heparin, platelets and antibiotics).

3. Broad-spectrum antimicrobials, e.g. cefuroxime i.v. (one dose pre-operatively and two doses post-operatively).
   - Endotoxin may be absorbed from intestine causing endotoxaemia and contributing to the renal failure seen post-operatively.
   - Bacteria from the biliary system (usually Gram-negative) may cause septicaemia or wound infection.

4. Nutritional support.
   - Malnourishment is corrected, total parenteral nutrition (TPN) in selected cases.
   - Aromatic amino acids may precipitate hepatic encephalopathy.

5. Bile salts, e.g. sodium deoxycholate.
   - May reduce endotoxin absorption from the intestine.
   - May reduce the risk of post-operative renal failure.

6. Biliary drainage.
   - Is indicated if serum bilirubin is very high, e.g. >155 μmol/L.
   - Reduces the risk of hepatic encephalopathy.

- (a) Endoscopic sphincterotomy (periampullary carcinoma, ascending cholangitis with calculous obstruction of the biliary tree) or (b) a stent (malignant biliary obstruction) which can be sited endoscopically or percutaneously may be used to drain bile.
- External percutaneous transhepatic drainage is associated with many complications, e.g. sepsis, haemobilia, fistulae, bile peritonitis, etc. and is not recommended.

7. Hepatitis serology should be performed on jaundiced patients undergoing surgery (especially hepatitis B) so that appropriate precautions are taken in infected cases.

PAPER III

QUESTIONS

Write short notes on:

1. Split-thickness skin autografts.
2. Treatment of early breast cancer.
3. Carpal tunnel syndrome.
4. The clinical presentation and management of benign prostatic hyperplasia.
5. The surgical implications of AIDS.
6. Slipped upper femoral epiphysis.
7. Post-operative DVT.
8. The indications for percutaneous transluminal angioplasty (PTA) and its complications.

ANSWERS

1. Split-thickness skin autografts

- These grafts contain the epidermis and a portion of the dermis. They can be further subclassified into thin, intermediate or thick.

Advantages
1. Grafts become vascularized rapidly.
2. Grafts survive well on less than ideal recipient sites, e.g. irradiated sites, contaminated wounds, burn surfaces, etc.
3. Donor sites heal rapidly and can be re-used within 10 days.

Disadvantages
1. Great tendency to contract. Rigid splints may be used in preventing contractures.
2. Colour and texture mismatch.
3. Impaired sensation.

4. Low resistance to trauma.

Donor sites

1. Commonly used sites include: thighs (inner medial); upper arm (medial); buttocks; abdominal wall and shaved scalp which may be used in large burns.
2. Donor sites heal by reepithelialization from the remains of the pilosebaceous units within 10–21 days.
3. A semipermeable membrane such as Opsite protects the donor site from trauma and dehydration.

Instruments for obtaining grafts

1. Knives, e.g. the Humby knife has an adjustable roller that controls the thickness of the graft.
2. Dermatomes.
   - Drum dermatomes (reliable thickness gauge).
   - Power-driven dermatomes save a great deal of time during grafting and can be used by the less experienced surgeon.

Notes

A. A special cutting machine may be used to create a mesh pattern out of split skin grafts.

B. The skin graft can be folded and wrapped in a swab soaked in normal saline in a sterile jar to be stored in a refrigerator for up to 20 days. Grafts can also be stored by applying them temporarily to the donor site.

Recipient sites

1. Recipient sites should have good vascularity, good haemostasis and low bacterial counts. Contaminated and non-viable tissue should be excised.
2. Good contact between the graft and the recipient bed is required.
3. A fibrin network develops between the graft and the recipient site during the first 48 hours through which plasmatic imbibition occurs. Vascular buds then grow into the fibrin network and the graft.
4. Grafts can be fixed with sutures, staples, tapes or adhesives.
5. Dressing methods of skin grafts include: tie-over dressing, pressure dressing epithelial inlay and the open method. The dressing is usually left undisturbed for 5–7 days.

Notes

1. Factors responsible for graft loss include infection (especially with S. pyogenes) and poor contact with the recipient bed (e.g. due to haematoma or seroma)
2. In thin grafts, the graft is more likely to survive and the donor site heals faster. However there is greater contraction and colour and texture mismatch.
3. Culture-derived keratinoycte sheets are now available.

---

2. Treatment of early breast cancer

Conservation surgery

- Partial mastectomy, in the form of lumpectomy or quadrantectomy, combined with an axillary dissection and followed by radiotherapy to the whole breast is the mainstay of management of early breast cancer. It has a disease-free survival and an overall survival equivalent to radical mastectomy.

Axillary disease

- Axillary dissection (levels I, II and III) is recommended in most patients except those with non-invasive carcinoma only or who have a previously irradiated axilla. Although axillary dissection is associated with a significant morbidity (lymphoedema of the arm, seroma, intercostobrachial neuralgia and stiff shoulder) and has no impact on survival, it has the advantage of determining the nodal status, the best single predictor of prognosis, and reducing the incidence of loco-regional recurrence.

Non-palpable cancer

- Screening mammography has grown rapidly due to the publication of data supporting its role in saving the lives of women.
- The localization with a straight needle or hook wire is performed by the radiologist, and the specimen is radiographed after excision to ensure an adequate removal of the mammographic abnormality.
- Ultrasound localization where applicable is the method of choice.
- Stereotactic localization is more accurate than other methods, and allows fine needle aspiration cytology to be performed. The role of the latter procedure is still unclear.
- Non-palpable cancers are smaller, more often node negative and are more likely to be non-invasive.

Mastectomy

- The current indications for mastectomy include multifocal disease, primary carcinoma >5 cm, centrally located carcinoma, recurrent carcinoma (within 5 years) and the express wish of the patient.
- Patey's mastectomy (total mastectomy combined with axillary dissection) is usually performed.
- Simple mastectomy is performed for multifocal non-invasive cancer or when mastectomy is indicated and the axilla was previously

irradiated.

Breast reconstruction (BR)

- BR should be offered to all patients who must undergo mastectomy. Textured silicone implants, tissue expanders, latissimus dorsi myocutaneous flap or the TRAM flap may be used.

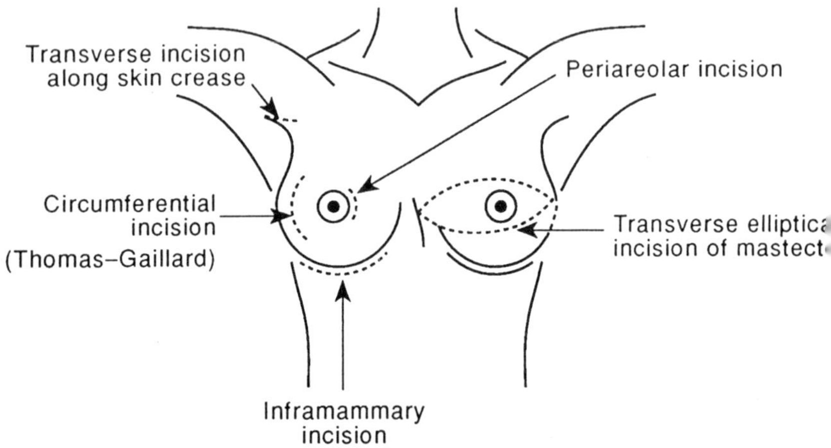

Figure Diagram demonstrating some breast surgery incisions

Tamoxifen

- All patients are prescribed tamoxifen 20 mg daily.
- The mechanism of action of this anti-oestrogen in breast cancer is still controversial, but it may be mediated by transformation growth factors secreted by the breast stroma.

Adjuvant systemic chemotherapy

- Fit patients with positive nodes or poorly differentiated carcinoma are selected for systemic chemotherapy of which various regimes are available, CMF, ECF, etc.

Psychological factors

- The role of the nurse counsellor is important.
- Establishing a good relationship between the surgical, medical,

radiotherapy and nursing team and the patient is conducive to successful management.

- Psychological morbidity associated with the diagnosis of breast cancer may need a psychiatric referral.

---

3. Carpal tunnel syndrome

Pathology

- The median nerve is compressed in the carpal tunnel under the flexor retinaculum.
- Commonest in middle-aged women.
- Causes include rheumatoid arthritis, osteoarthritis of the wrist, Colles' fractures, pregnancy, hypothyroidism, shoulder immobilization, acromegaly, diabetes mellitus, amyloidosis and fluid retaining drugs. Many cases are idiopathic.

Symptoms

- Tingling and paraesthesiae along median nerve distribution in the hand (the palmar aspect of the lateral three and a half fingers).
- Burning pain (worse at night) radiating into the forearm.
- Clumsiness in fine hand movements.

Signs

- Vary according to the severity and duration of compression.
- Sensory impairment along median nerve distribution in the hand.
- Partial wasting of thenar muscles.
- Motor weakness of median-innervated muscles (e.g. abductor pollicis brevis).
- Tinel sign (gentle tapping over the median nerve at wrist causes paraesthesiae).
- Phalen sign.

Investigations

Electrophysiological tests may show a conduction delay in the affected part of median nerve.

Differential diagnosis

Includes cervical rib, neuritis of median nerve, cervical spondylitis and other lesions of spinal cord, cervical root and brachial plexus.

Treatment

1. Conservative measures are tried first. They include a simple wrist splint and local steroid injection (10 mg hydrocortisone made up to 1 ml with 1% lignocaine is injected lateral to the midline of the volar aspect of the wrist).

2. Surgery. The flexor retinaculum is longitudinally divided and the median nerve is completely exposed. The motor branch to the thenar muscle and the palmar cutaneous branch should be avoided. The procedure can be performed via a curved incision parallel and ulnar to the thenar crease. At the level of the flexor wrist crease, the incision is angled towards the ulnar side. Division of the transverse ligament can be also achieved endoscopically using the two-portal technique. The latter procedure has the obvious advantage of minimizing scarring and wound complications.
   - Surgery is resorted to when conservative measures have failed or the condition is too advanced (e.g. wasting of abductor brevis).

---

4. The clinical presentation and management of benign prostatic hyperplasia (BPH)

This benign tumour of the periurethral prostatic tissue affects about 75% of men over the age of 80.

History

Poor urinary stream, urgency, frequency, hesitancy of micturition, symptoms of UTI, acute urinary retention (severe suprapubic pain with constant urgency), haematuria and overflow incontinence with chronic urinary retention. BPH may occur with no symptoms.

Examination

- An enlarged bladder due to urinary retention.
- Digital rectal examination may reveal an enlarged and smooth prostate with obliterated median sulcus.

Investigation

- MSU (microscopy and microbiology).
- FBC, plasma U + Es and creatinine.
- Serum PSA (prostatic specific antigen).
- Ultrasound of kidneys, ureters, bladder and prostate. Post-micturition urine volume can be estimated.
- An intravenous pyelogram (IVP) may show hydronephrosis, bladder calculi, trabeculations and diverticula. It is not performed routinely.
- Urodynamic studies. A high intravesical pressure and low urinary flow rate are common findings. They are indicated if there are marked irritative symptoms with little or no obstructive symptoms.

Differential diagnosis

Neurogenic bladder, bladder neck stenosis, prostatitis, urethral strictures and prostatic carcinoma.

Treatment

1. Acute urinary retention is relieved by catheterization (transurethral or suprapubic).
2. UTI is treated with appropriate antimicrobial therapy if there is evidence of systemic toxicity.
3. Chronic urinary retention. Catheterization is performed if there is renal impairment. Post-obstructive diuresis may ensue and i.v.

hydration may be required. Periodic clamping of the catheter is ineffective in stopping the haematuria which occasionally occurs. Any infection should be treated.

4. Surgical treatment. Indications include: very distressing symptoms; significant residual urine; persistent infection and secondary complications, such as renal impairment, bladder diverticula and calculi. Renal impairment should be corrected pre-operatively and monitored peri-operatively.
   a) TURP
      - Most commonly performed operation.
      - Lower rate of morbidity and mortality and shorter hospital stay than with open prostatectomy.
      - TUR syndrome (due to absorption of irrigating fluid) and retrograde ejaculation (75% of cases) are specific complications.
      - Relief of symptoms occurs in 95% of cases.
   b) Open prostatectomy (transvesical, retropubic or transperineal) is indicated for very large prostates (>60 g), when bladder complications (calculi and diverticula) are present and when positioning the patient for TURP is not possible for orthopaedic reasons.

5. Conservative treatment is indicated for symptomatic patients unfit for surgery or awaiting surgery.
   a) Permanent drainage with a Silastic catheter.
   b) α-Adrenergic blockers have been used to relieve symptoms with limited success, e.g. prazosin, indoramine.
   c) 5-Reductase inhibitors. Finasteride (Proscar) is effective in relieving symptoms, but takes a few months to show any benefit.
   d) Endoprostatic stent insertion.

5. The surgical implications of AIDS

For the surgeon and the operating room

- Risk of seroconversion following a needlestick injury is less than 0.5%.
- At-risk patients should be treated as HIV-positive.
- Gloves and eye protection should be worn for endoscopic procedures.
- AIDs specimens are clearly labelled and double bagged in impermeable bags. Gloves and gowns are used when handling specimens.
- Operating room and laboratory staff are notified prior to the procedure.
- All non-disposable items and work surfaces are decontaminated with freshly prepared 1:5 dilution of 5.25% sodium hypochlorite.
- In theatres, the number of staff should be reduced to a minimum and unnecessary equipment should be removed.
- The operating table is covered with a sheet of polythene, double gloves are worn and an attempt is made to use scissors and diathermy instead of scalpel for dissection.
- Instruments are autoclaved before being unpacked, then re-packed and re-autoclaved.
- Patient is allowed to recover in the operating room and not taken to the recovery room.

For the patient

- Screening blood donations does not exclude HIV transmission as the HIV-antibodies are screened for and not HIV-antigen.
- At-risk health workers should not be allowed to perform invasive procedures within patients' open tissues.
- Pre-operative nutritional support in malnourished HIV-infected patients may reduce post-operative complications.

Surgical referrals of HIV-infected patients

1. Anal warts.
   - More extensive than in HIV-negative patients.
   - Increased incidence of neoplastic transformation (especially HPV 16).
   - Electrocautery and lasers are used for eradication.
   - Podophyllin and topical 5-fluorouracil cream may be used.

2. Peri-anal sepsis.
   - Herpes simplex (HSV) and *Mycobacterium avium intracellulare* may be responsible.

3. Anal ulceration.
   - Virology swabs are taken (HSV and CMV).
   - There may be associated diarrhoea (stool microscopy and culture).
   - Rectal biopsies for CMV and *Cryptosporidium*.
   - Lymphoma and Kaposi's sarcoma may cause ulceration.

4. Abdominal pain.
   - Opportunistic infections especially with CMV and *Cryptosporidium*.
   - Infiltration of liver and spleen with lymphoma or *Mycobacterium avium intracellulare* may cause jaundice and rarely abdominal pain.
   - Bowel obstruction may be caused by lymphoma or atypical mycobacteria.
   - Bowel perforation may be caused by CMV infection.

5. Lymph node biopsy.

6. Splenectomy for thrombocytopenic purpura.

7. Insertion of Hickman lines.

---

6. Slipped upper femoral epiphysis

Pathology
- The femoral shaft moves proximally and rotates externally (the usual mechanism). Occasionally it is the femoral epiphysis which moves relative to the acetabulum.
- Age group usually affected 10–20 years.
- Commoner in males.
- Associated with an endocrine abnormality in about 40% of cases, e.g. obesity, hypothyroidism, tall stature, sexual immaturity, etc.
- Also associated with Marfan's syndrome, scurvy, renal rickets and local radiotherapy.
- History of trauma is present in about 35% of cases.

Clinical features
- Limp.
- Pain in the groin, hip or knee.
- The affected limb may be shortened and externally rotated.
- Features due to endocrine abnormalities.

Radiographs
- The AP film of the hip may appear normal.
- It is essential to have a lateral film of the hip. The epiphysis appears to have tilted backwards and downwards. The angle of the displacement can be measured (see Figure).

Classification

A. Acute.
   - Recent history of sudden onset of limp and pain.
   - No new bone formation is seen.

B. Acute-on-chronic.
   - Long-standing history of symptoms with sudden exacerbation.
   - Little new bone formation is noted on the radiographs.

C. Chronic.
   - Long-standing history of symptoms.
   - New bone formation is seen.

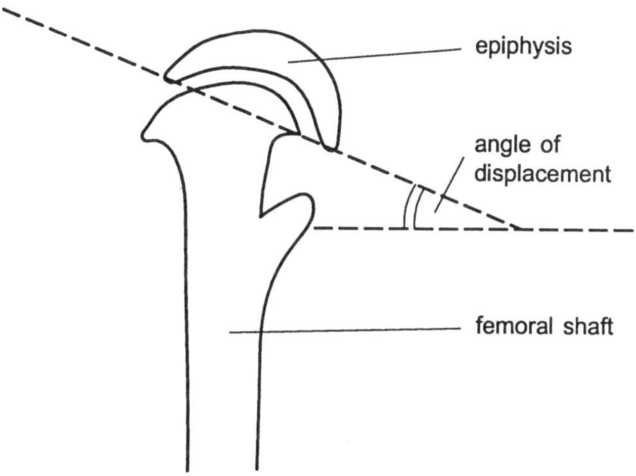

Treatment

1. Acute and acute-on-chronic cases.
   - If the angle of displacement is <35° the epiphysis should be pinned. Moore's pins, Nystrium nails and AO screws are suitable devices.
   - If the slip is >35°, gentle reduction under GA is attempted (traction in the mid-abduction/abduction range and internal rotation). If the angle becomes <35° the epiphysis is pinned, but if the angle remains >35° operative reduction is indicated where the greater trochanter is detached to facilitate the reduction.

2. Chronic cases.
   - If the slip is <35° the epiphysis is pinned.
   - If the slip is >35° then a subtrochanteric osteotomy is a suitable operation. A plate or spica is used until the osteotomy is united.

Complications

1. Avascular necrosis of the epiphysis.
   - The risk of this complication is reduced by early diagnosis, gentle handling of the epiphysis and surrounding tissue during operative procedures, and avoiding forceful manipulation and unsuitable devices.

- In an established case osteotomy or arthroplasty may be considered.

2. Osteoarthritis.

3. Slipped upper femoral epiphysis on the other side. The opposite hip should always be checked and followed up in patients affected by this condition. Only 1 in 5 of these patients has a strictly normal contralateral hip.

---

7. Post-operative DVT

Pathogenesis

Virchow's triad:
[Changes in the vessel walls
[Flow stasis
[Hypercoagulability

Risk factors
These include: obesity, cardiac disease, previous DVT, hip and pelvic operations, pregnancy, anaemia, polycythaemia, old age (>60), varicose veins, oestrogen-containing oral contraceptive pill, malignancy and hemiplegia.

Clinical features
1. Symptoms and signs may be absent.
2. Pain and tightness in the calf or thigh.
3. Swelling of the limb.
4. Phlegmasia alba dolens and phlegmasia caerulea dolens may develop if the ileo-femoral segment is involved.
5. Fever and tachycardia.
6. Homan's sign may be present.
7. Pulmonary embolism.

Differential diagnosis
1. Rupture of calf muscle fibres especially in out-of-condition athletes.
2. Rupture of popliteal synovial cysts.
3. Kaposi's sarcoma of the lower leg in AIDS patients.

Investigations
1. Ascending venography.
   - The most accurate investigation, detecting about 95% of cases.
   - Radioisotopes have been recently introduced to replace contrast media.
2. Doppler scanning.
   - Inexpensive, non-invasive and can be repeated frequently.
   - Insensitive to calf vein thrombosis but has good accuracy (90%) in detecting thrombosis proximal to the popliteal system.
3. Radioactive fibrinogen.
   - Time consuming.
   - Requires isotope source.

   - Useless in detecting DVTs in the common femoral and iliac veins.
4. Plethysmography.
   This is an excellent investigation especially in high ileo-femoral DVT where sensitivity is about 96% and specificity is about 99%.

Complications
1. Pulmonary embolism.
2. Venous gangrene.
3. Chronic venous insufficiency.
4. Varicose veins.

Prophylaxis
1. Heparin.
   - Most widely used in prophylaxis.
   - 5000 IU subcutaneously twice daily starting 2 hours pre-operatively.
   - Reduces incidence of DVT from about 25% to about 7%.
   - New preparations include low molecular weight form and a combination with dihydroergotamine.
2. Dextran 70.
3. Antiplatelet drugs (aspirin, dipyridamole).
4. Ancrod.
5. Graded pressure elastic stockings, e.g. TED stockings.
6. Intermittent pneumatic compression of the calf.
7. Active leg exercises, leg elevation and early mobilization.

Treatment of DVT
1. Bed rest, elevation and elastic support.
2. Full anticoagulation (unless contra-indicated) with heparin initially (APTT ~1.5–2 times control) followed by warfarin for at least 3 months (monitored by INR).
3. Fibrinolytic agents, e.g. streptokinase and urokinase.

---

8. The indications for percutaneous transluminal angioplasty (PTA) and its complications

Indications

1. Peripheral vascular disease. Stenoses or short occlusions (<10 cm long) of the common iliac, external iliac, common femoral, superficial femoral or popliteal arteries can be treated with PTA. The one year success rate declines from proximal to distal, being 85% for common iliac disease, 70% for external iliac disease, and 50% for femoral and popliteal arteries.
   PTA is contraindicated if
   a) the occlusion is long (>10 cm)
   b) no aterial lumen is visualized distal to the obstruction
   c) the artery is blocked flush with its origin.

2. Renal artery stenosis. The one year success rate is 60% for fibromuscular dysplasia (90% is the immediate success rate). The results are not as good for atherosclerosis.

3. Coronary artery disease. PTA is indicated if
   a) there is severe symptoms associated with a single vessel disease or mild double vessel disease
   b) the patient is high risk for operation, e.g. acute myocardial infarction, cardiogenic shock, etc.

4. Other indications include intestinal angina due to mesenteric vascular disease. Budd–Chiari syndrome, occluded porto-caval anastomsis in portal hypertension, etc.

Complications of PTA

1. At the site of arterial puncture:
   a) haematoma.
   b) haemorrhage.
   c) false aneurysm.
   These complications can be avoided or reduced by applying adequate pressure at the site of arterial puncture after removing the angioplasty catheter.

2. At the site of angioplasty:
   a) arterial rupture (due to balloon or guide wire) .

b) aneurysm formation.
c) subintimal arterial dissection.
d) recurrence of arterial obstruction. The rate depends upon the site and cause of obstruction. Antiplatelet drugs may reduce the incidence.

3. Within the vasculature distal to the angioplasty site:
a) embolisation – the incidence is 5%.
b) thrombosis.
c) arterial spasm.

PAPER IV

QUESTIONS

Write short notes on:

1. The causes and treatment of an acutely ischaemic limb.
2. The initial management of the burned patient.
3. The causes, diagnosis and treatment of paralytic ileus.
4. The role of medical imaging in the assessment of blunt abdominal trauma.
5. Screening for colorectal cancer.
6. Post-operative wound infection.
7. Total parenteral nutrition.
8. Cervical rib.

ANSWERS

1. The causes and treatment of an acutely ischaemic limb

Causes

1. Embolus – the heart is the source of embolus in 85% of cases.
   - The embolus may originate from the left atrium in patients with atrial fibrillation or from mural thrombus in patients with myocardial infarction.
   - Prosthetic valves, infective endocarditis (septic emboli), aneurysms (aortic, iliac, femoral and popliteal), cardiac tumours and venous thrombi migrating through a patent foramen ovale (paradoxic emboli) are recognised sources of emboli.
   - Distal embolisation complicates 5% of transluminal angioplasty procedures.

2. Thrombosis
   - Haemorrhagic dissection beneath an atherosclerotic plaque is the

usual mechanism of acute thrombotic occlusion in patients with peripheral vascular disease.
- History and clinical examination may help to differentiate between embolus and thrombosis as a cause of acute arterial occlusion.

3. Trauma.
   Traumatic causes include:
   a) fractures, e.g. fracture of the shaft of femur may injure the superficial femoral artery
   b) dislocations, e.g. posterior dislocation of the knee may injure the popliteal artery
   c) blunt trauma
   d) penetrating injury
   e) crushing injury
   f) traction injury
   g) chemical injury, e.g. intraarterial injection of a sclerosant injury
   h) iatragenic, e.g. angioplasty, inadvertent ligation or division of an artery.

Principles of management
1. Thrombosis and embolism.
   a) Immediate anticoagulation by intravenous heparin in order to slow the propagation of thrombus and allow time for the assessment of collateral circulation and preparation for surgery if indicated.
   b) Fogarty catheter embolectomy or thrombectomy. The catheter is inserted through a proximal arteriotomy (e.g. the common femoral artery). Intraoperative infusion of a thrombolytic agent may be used in conjunction with embolectomy when thrombus has propagated.
   c) Intra-arterial infusion of a thrombolytic agent (such as urokinase, streptokinase or tPA) may restore patency in thrombotic occlusion.
   d) Open thrombectomy (±vein patch).
   e) Percutaneous transluminal angioplasty (PTA) may be used to recanalise short thrombotic occlusions
   f) Arterial reconstruction with synthetic or autogenous venous grafts may be required if the ischaemia is still reversible and the above methods have failed.

g) Amputation is indicated if irreversible ischaemia has supervened.
h) Fasciotomy may be required in order to prevent or treat compartment syndrome.
i) Reperfusion syndrome should be treated with hydration and alkalinization of urine.

2. Trauma. The principles include
   a) resuscitation and control of haemorrhage
   b) systemic heparinization
   c) exploration of penetrating injuries
   d) closure of arterial lacerations (± vein patch)
   e) Fogarty catheter thrombectomy
   f) excision of severely damaged arterial segments and end-to-end anastomosis if possible after mobilization of artery, if direct anastomosis is not possible then an autogenous vein graft is used to allow revascularization
   g) local application of papaverine for arterial spasm
   h) fasciotomy
   i) ampulation for irreversible ischaemia or failure of revascularisation
   j) tetanus and antibiotic cover
   k) reduction and stabilizations of fractures and dislocations.

---

2. The initial management of the burned patient

1. Remove the burning source: electrical, thermal, chemical or ionizing radiation.

2. Ensure adequate airway and breathing.
   - Endotracheal intubation may be required if laryngeal oedema is present.
   - Humidified oxygen via a face mask is indicated in all cases of suspected inhaled gases or smoke.
   - Pulmonary oedema may necessitate mechanical ventilation.

3. Place the injured area in a cold bath or under running cold water. Phenol burns are an exception as water accelerates the absorption of phenol. In this situation, polyethylene glycol is used.

4. Assess the depth and surface area of burns.
   - Full-thickness burns appear as insensitive dry white areas, whereas partial-thickness burns appear as sensitive red areas.
   - For calculation of surface area the rule of nines is used.

5. Cover the burns with a sterile dressing.

6. Fluid resuscitation.
   - Various formulae have been devised. Dextran 110, HPPF and Ringer's lactate are commonly used.
   - i.v. Fluid replacement is necessary in burns >10% in children and >15% in adults.
   - For adults (70 kg) – 125 ml of HPPF per 10% surface area burned over first 24 hours. 50% of that is given in the first 8 hours and the other half is given over the following 16 hours.
   - For children – 45 ml of HPPF per kg per 15% surface area burned. 50% in the first 8 hours and the other half in the following 16 hours.
   - Circulatory volume should be monitored during resuscitation by pulse, blood pressure, urine output, serum U + Es, haematocrit and central venous pressure.

7. Pain control.
   - Adequate analgesia is essential.
   - Analgesic requirements vary from opiates (low dose i.v. or infusion pump), to oral or rectal paracetamol. Dihydrocodeine may be given for intermediate pain. Self-administered Entonox has proved useful in pain control.

8. Tetanus prophylaxis is given as indicated.

9. Systemic antibiotics.
   - Routine use is not recommended as it encourages the emergence of resistant strains and colonization by yeasts and fungi.
   - Antibiotics commonly used include penicillin (for group A streptococci), flucloxacillin (for *Staphylococcus aureus*) and gentamicin (for Gram-negative septicaemia).
   - Toxic shock syndrome should be diagnosed early and treated promptly.

10. Divide any constricting eschars longitudinally.

11. Wound management.
    - Combination of exposure (for facial and perianal burns) and closed dressing techniques. In the closed technique 1% silver sulphadiazine is applied to the wound which is then covered by absorptive dressings. Aseptic techniques are used.

---

3. The causes, diagnosis and treatment of paralytic ileus

Definition

Failure of peristalsis of the intestine due to neuromuscular inhibition. It may be segmental or generalized.

Causes

1. Intra-abdominal inflammation, e.g. generalized peritonitis, pancreatitis, acute appendicitis (segmental).
2. Metabolic disorders, e.g. hypokalaemia, uraemia of renal failure, diabetic ketoacidosis, hypomagnesaemia.
3. Reflex sympathetic overactivity, e.g. handling of intestine during surgery, multiple trauma.
4. Drugs, e.g. ganglion-blocking drugs.
5. Septicaemia.
6. Neurogenic (seen in spinal cord damage, retroperitoneal haematoma).
7. Vascular ischaemia of the intestine.
8. Hirschsprung's disease is a form of regional ileus.

Clinical features

1. Features of the underlying condition.
2. Abdominal pain is usually absent. However, it is occasionally seen.
3. Effortless vomiting (not faeculent).
4. Abdominal distension.
5. No passage of flatus PR 48 hours after laparatomy.
6. Dehydration (not characteristic).
7. Bowel sounds are usually absent.
8. Abdominal radiographs show gas throughout the intestine (cf. in mechanical bowel obstruction gas is seen up to the point of obstruction only).

Treatment

1. Correction of fluid and electrolyte imbalance, especially potassium and urea.
2. Nasogastric tube to relieve distension and vomiting. NG tube should not be spigoted.
3. Treatment of underlying cause.
4. NBM until the patient passes flatus PR then sips of water are started and oral intake is gradually built towards normal diet.

Notes

- Paralytic ileus usually settles down in 2–4 days.
- The risk and severity of postoperative paralytic ileus can be reduced by gentle handling of intestine at operation.

---

4. The role of medical imaging in the assessment of blunt abdominal trauma

Plain radiography

Plain radiographs still play an important role:

1. Fractures of the lumbar spine and pelvis are easily seen on plain radiographs.
2. Signs of free intraperitoneal gas include:
   a) Visualization of the falciform ligament of the liver.
   b) Visualization of the under-surface of the hemidiaphragms.
   c) Visualization of the lateral wall of the large bowel (due to collection of gas in the paracolic gutters).
3. Dilatation of the small and large intestine down to the rectum may indicate paralytic ileus due to trauma.
4. Localized dilatation of small intestine may indicate an injury to a neighbouring organ, e.g. pancreas.
5. Alteration of solid organs outline may suggest organ damage.
6. Loss of psoas shadow may be associated with retroperitoneal injury.

Plain radiography after the administration of contrast media has a role in the assessment of urological trauma, e.g. cystogram for bladder rupture, IVU for renal injuries.

CT Scan

- Indicated if organ damage is suspected.
- Oral and i.v. contrast media increase pick-up rate.
- Sections should include the lower parts of the pelvis where collections may be found in the pouch of Douglas.
- CT has replaced angiography and scintigraphy in the assessment of vascular and solid organ injuries.
- Injury to solid organs such as liver, spleen, pancreas and kidneys is easily detected.
- Fresh intraperitoneal blood appears dense on CT scanning. Hounsfield units are used to quantify density, e.g. 24 H. units for fresh blood. The density gradually decreases with time and after 48–72 hours it reaches that of water and appears similar to ascites on CT scanning.
- CT scan, when available, has many advantages over urography in the assessment of renal injuries:
  a) It is more accurate.
  b) It allows grading of injury, e.g. contusion, cortical laceration, etc.

c) It gives faster result.
d) It requires less manipulation of the patient.
e) It involves less radiation.

- Peritoneal lavage is more sensitive than CT scanning in detecting small intraperitoneal bleeds. However, the small haemorrhages detected by peritoneal lavage will invariably lead to unnecessary laparatomy (if CT is not used).
- Disadvantages of CT scanning are:
  a) Requires more cooperation from the patient than with ultrasound (US).
  b) Equipment is not portable (cf. ultrasound).

Ultrasound

- Indicated if solid organ injury is suspected.
- Useful in detecting solid organ injury and intraperitoneal bleeding.
- Advantages:
  a) Portable.
  b) Cheap.
  c) Requires less cooperation from the patient who may be very ill, compared with CT scanning.
  d) Quick to perform.
- Disadvantages:
  a) Imaging may be impaired by gas (ileus) or bone.
  b) Drains and dressing may interfere with imaging.
  c) Less accurate than CT scanning in detecting solid organ damage.

Magnetic resonance imaging (MRI)

- MRI has no role (at present) in abdominal trauma due to technical unavailability.

Angiography and scintigraphy

- Have been gradually replaced by CT scanning.
- Scintigraphy may be superior to CT in detecting small leaks, e.g. from biliary system.
- Scintigraphy is useful in the follow-up assessment of organ function, e.g. kidney function after renal trauma.

---

5. Screening for colorectal cancer

High risk groups include patients with:
1. Ulcerative colitis.
2. Familial polyposis coli.
3. Previous history of colonic cancer.
4. Muir syndrome.
5. Peutz-Jegher syndrome.
6. Family cancer syndrome.
7. Crohn disease.
8. Ureterosigmoidostomy.
9. Turcot's syndrome.
10. Gardner's syndrome.

The risk also increases with age.

Methods of screening
1. Digital rectal examination.
   Only 10% of colorectal cancers are within the reach of this method.
   Low pick-up rate.

2. Proctosigmoidoscopy.
   The flexible sigmoidoscope has a higher pick-up rate (about 2.5 times greater) and covers a longer distance (60 cm vs 20 cm) than the rigid sigmoidoscope. It is particularly useful for screening patients with ureterosigmoidostomy.

3. Colonoscopy.
   Particularly suitable for screening patients with ulcerative colitis (for more than 10 years), previous resection of colorectal cancer and with hereditary bowel cancer. Multiple biopsies may be taken.

4. Faecal occult blood (FOB) testing.
   The most widely used screening test (it may not be cost-effective due to low yield). Several tests are available:
   a) Haemoccult test:
      i) Principle:
      Phenolic compounds + H_2O_2 → quinone compounds (blue)
      ↑ haemoglobin or peroxidases

- ii) False positive results can be produced by diet (red meat, carrots, etc.), drugs (ferrous sulphate), delayed processing of slides and povidone iodine contamination.
- iii) Rate of cancer detection = 3/1000.
- iv) Rate of false positives = 25%.
- v) Six specimens from two different parts of three consecutive stools are usually tested.
- vi) A peroxidase inhibitor may be added to the reagent.

b) Immunological methods:
- Specific antibody to human haemoglobin is used to detect occult faecal blood.
- Various techniques used: immunofluorescence, radial immunodiffusion, counter immunoelectrophoresis and ELISA.

c) Hemo quant.

faecal haem (non-fluorescent) → porphyrin (fluorescent) (fluorometry)

A positive FOB test is an indication for a thorough history and examination, sigmoidoscopy and colonoscopy.

5. Cancer markers.
   - a) Carcinoembryonic antigen (CEA). Serial plasma levels are useful in screening for recurrence.
   - b) Faecal lithocholic/deoxycholic acid ratio.
   - c) DNA of colonic biopsies may be analysed by flow cytometry.
   - d) Monosialoganglioside antigen (detection of recurrence).

Success of screening programmes depends on:
- i) False positives.
- ii) False negatives.
- iii) Cost-effectiveness.
- iv) Effect on survival.

6. Post-operative wound infection

Classification of surgical wounds

- Class I (clean wounds) e.g. thyroid surgery. Infection rate is less than 2%. Infection is usually exogenous with *Staphylococcus* being the commonest causative organism.

- Class II (clean-contaminated). The GI and respiratory tracts are entered during an elective operation with minimal spillage of contents, e.g. cholecystectomy. Infection rate is around 7%.

- Class III (contaminated) as in II but with excessive spillage of contents, and where there is an obvious infection, e.g. appendicectomy in acute appendicitis. Infection rate around 18%.

- Class IV (dirty wounds) where there is pus or GI tract perforation. Infection rate is around 40%.

- Infections in classes II, III and IV are usually due to endogenous bacteria.

Types of wound infections

1. Minor superficial wound infection presents with local pain, erythema, discharge and/or pyrexia. Staphylococci and streptococci are usually responsible.
2. Cellulitis.
3. Abcess.

Factors influencing wound infection

1. Bacterial factors: type, virulence and dose.
2. Local wound factors: wound class, oxygen tension, blood supply, haematoma, necrotic tissue, foreign body, etc.
3. Patient factors (phagocytosis, neutrophil function, opsonization).
   - Immunosuppression: congenital immunodeficiency syndrome, AIDS, diabetes, drugs (corticosteroids, cytotoxins, etc.), malignancy, debilitating illness.
   - Nutrition.
4. Theatre asepsis.
5. Surgical technique in handling tissue and wound closure (gentle handling of tissue, tapes and staples give a lower infection rate than

sutures (no tension on sutures).

6. Duration of hospitalization (pre- and post-operative): if prolonged, infection rate may increase.
7. Pre-operative removal of hair at the operative site with depilatory cream on the day of operation decreases the infection rate. Razor shaving the day before may increase the infection rate.
8. Duration of operation. The longer the duration, the higher the infection rate.
9. The presence of a remote source of infection increases the infection rate.
10. The use of prophylactic antimicrobials (type, dose, route and timing should be appropriately chosen).
11. Prophylactic use of surgical drains may increase the infection rate.

Treatment of infected wounds

- Once a wound is clearly infected, the sutures should be removed.
- Pus must be drained.
- Slough and devitalized tissue are removed by surgical debridement or by topical preparations (e.g. dextranomer, streptodornase, etc.).
- Infected wounds which are properly cleaned can be closed with tapes or loose sutures rather than waiting for healing by secondary intention.
- Heavily contaminated wounds are cleaned and packed for 5–7 days and once clean can be closed by delayed primary closure or allowed to heal by secondary intention.
- Cellulitis is treated with appropriate antibiotics after taking a swab for culture and sensitivity.
- Skin grafting may be necessary.

---

7. Total parenteral nutrition (TPN)

Indications

1. Short bowel syndrome.
2. Gastrointestinal fistulae (TPN helps healing and closure).
3. Severe and recurrent pancreatitis.
4. Hypercatabolic states, e.g. major trauma, severe burns, sepsis.
5. Crohn's disease of the small bowel.
6. Severe mucositis of the intestine following chemotherapy.
7. Pre-operative nutritional build-up of malnourished patients undergoing surgery.
8. Intestinal obstruction and paralytic ileus are recognized indications.
9. Radiation enteritis.
10. Liver failure.
11. Anorexia nervosa.

Nutrient requirements

- Vary widely, influenced by age, extent of malnutrition and disease activity.
- Calories are provided by carbohydrates (glucose, sorbitol and fructose) and/or fat emulsions. Usual requirements 2000–3000 kcal.
- Fluid requirements are decreased in hepatic, cardiac and renal failure but increased in patients with high output fistulae or large nasogastric aspirate. Average daily requirement is about 2500–3000 ml.
- Nitrogen (N) requirement is about 15 g N for an adult. Essential amino acids must be provided.
- Electrolytes such as Na^+, K^+, Ca^{2+}, Mg^{2+}, phosphate, are required daily.
- Various vitamins (e.g. vitamin C, D, K, B-complex) are required.
- Some trace elements are required daily.
- Hyperosmolar solutions should be administered via a central line. The line is usually inserted through the subclavian vein (infra-clavicular approach) and the tip lies in the superior vena cava (SVC).

Monitoring

6 hourly:	Pulse, temperature and respiratory rate.
Daily:	Serum urea, Na^+, K^+, glucose, Ca^{2+} and phosphate, haematocrit, body weight (an increase >0.3 kg/day

	indicates fluid retention and accurate fluid charts are required).
Once weekly:	Serum, zinc and magnesium.
Twice weekly:	Liver function tests.

Complications

1. Catheter problems: pneumothorax, air embolism, thrombophlebitis, thrombosis, PE, cardiac tamponade, damage to brachial plexus, brachial artery or thoracic duct, sepsis.
2. Hyperosmolarity–hyperglycaemia syndrome.
3. Hyperlipidaemia.
4. Electrolyte disturbance.
5. Glucose intolerance (insulin may be required).
6. Liver dysfunction.
7. Essential fatty acid deficiency.
8. Lactic acidosis.
9. Vitamin and trace elements deficiency.
10. Acalculous cholecystitis.

8. Cervical rib

Pathology

- An overdevelopment of the costal process of C7.
- Present in about 0.5% of population.
- Bilateral in about 50% of cases. Commoner on the right.
- Damage to the subclavian artery and lowest trunk of the brachial plexus as they arch over the rib produces the symptoms.

Symptoms (often absent)

A. Neurological. Pain and paraesthesiae in the forearm and hand (mainly on the ulnar side). Clumsiness in the fine movement of the hand.

B. Vascular. Varies from gangrene of fingers to mild cyanosis of the hand.

Signs

- Sensory impairment related to lowest trunk distribution.
- Muscle wasting (thenar, hypothenar and interossei).
- Weak or absent radial pulse with signs of ischaemia.

Investigations

Radiographs: Oblique views of the thoracic inlet demonstrate the cervical rib.

Arteriography: This may reveal constriction of the subclavian artery with post-stenotic dilatation.

Differential diagnosis

1. First rib syndrome.
2. Prolapsed intervertebral disc at C7–T1.
3. Peripheral lesions of median and ulnar nerves (neuritis, compression).
4. Spinal cord lesions (syringomyelia, tumours, poliomyelitis, etc.).
5. Pancoast tumour.
6. Raynaud's disease.

Treatment

1. Physiotherapy is employed in mild cases to strengthen the tone of girdle elevators.

2. Surgery is recommended for severe symptoms and signs and progressive cases. The scalenus anterior is divided. If this does not release the compressed structures, then the scalenus medius is divided and the cervical rib is resected. Occlusion of the subclavian artery may be treated with vascular reconstruction using a vein graft.

PAPER V

QUESTIONS

Write short notes on:

1. The principles of transplantation and rejection.
2. Complications of total hip arthroplasty.
3. The indications for surgery and surgical treatment of duodenal ulceration.
4. Surgical options for ulcerative colitis.
5. Surgical audit.
6. Diagnostic peritoneal lavage.
7. The clinical features and treatment of meconium ileus
8. Hazards of blood transfusion.

ANSWERS

1. The principles of transplantation and rejection

Transplantation antigens

- Major transplantation antigens are glycoproteins present on the surface of nucleated cells. They are known as human leukocyte-associated (HLA) antigens.
- HLA antigens are coded for by the major histocompatibility complex (MHC) carried on the short arm of the 6th chromosome in humans.
- MHC loci are designated as A, B, C and D. A, B and C code for class I antigens whereas D locus codes for class II antigens.
- Tissue typing is carried out by incubating the individual's lymphocytes with standard typing antisera or more recently by using monoclonal antibodies.
- Matching at A, B and DR loci is more crucial to the transplant survival than at other loci.
- ABO compatibility is essential for all transplants.

Graft rejection

A. Afferent phase. T cells are sensitized by:
   i) Antigen presenting dendritic cells (within the graft).
   ii) Recipient's macrophages which come in contact with graft antigens.
   iii) Interleukin-I secreted by macrophages. Sensitized CD4 cells release Interleukin-II. CD4 cells also secrete interleukin-I.

B. Efferent phase involves CD4 cells, CD8 cells (cytotoxic), cytokines, cytotoxic macrophages and antibodies (produced by activated B cells).
   - Class II antigens are more potent sensitizers than class I antigens.

1. Hyperacute rejection.
   - Antibody mediated.
   - Preformed antibodies are caused by previous blood transfusions, pregnancy and previous failed transplants.
   - Usually occurs within hours of transplantation.
   - Treated by removal of transplant.

2. Accelerated rejection.
   - Seen about 3 days post-transplantation.

3. Acute rejection.
   - Usually occurs within 3 months of transplantation.
   - Cell-mediated process involving CD4 cells, CD8 cells and cytokines.
   - May present with mild pyrexia, swelling and deterioration in function of the graft.
   - Diagnosis is established by graft biopsy, duplex doppler blood flow or isotope scanning.
   - Treated with corticosteroids and anti-lymphocyte preparations.

4. Chronic rejection.
   - Seen 1–4 years post-transplantation.
   - Presents with gradual deterioration in graft function.
   - Immunological mechanism unknown.
   - Ureteric obstruction and late development of hypertension should prompt a search for renal artery stenosis and rejection-mediated accelerated atherosclerosis.

Methods of immunosuppression

1. Cyclosporin A.
   - 11 amino acid fungal metabolite.
   - Inhibits the transcription of the genes coding for certain cytokines, e.g. IL-2, γ-IF.
2. Corticosteroids, e.g. prednisolone.
   - Block the release of IL-1, cause T-cell lymphopenia.
3. Azathioprine.
   - Metabolized to 6-mercaptopurine which acts as an anti-metabolite which reduces lymphocyte proliferation.
4. Cyclophosphamide.
   - Alkylating metabolites cause cross-links between DNA strands thus inhibiting lymphocyte proliferation.
5. Anti-T cell monoclonal antibodies.
6. Anti-lymphocyte globulins.
7. Irradiation.
8. Thoracic duct fistula.
9. Thymectomy.
10. Plasmapheresis.

Complications of immunosuppression

1. Increased incidence of infection – bacterial, viral, fungal and protozoal.
2. Increased incidence of malignancy, e.g. lymphoma, skin melanoma.
3. Complications specific to the immunosuppressive agent, e.g. nephrotoxicity (cyclosporin), osteoporosis (steroids).

---

2. Complications of total hip arthroplasty

Early complications

1. DVT and pulmonary embolism.
   - Without prophylaxis the incidence of DVT may be as high as 70% and PE as high as 20%.
   - Prophylactic methods include: heparin (subcutaneously 5000 IU bd), TED stockings, dextran infusion, low-dose warfarin, anti-thrombin III (combined with heparin), inflatable calf compressors and the recently-introduced low molecular weight heparin.
   - Regional anaesthesia has reduced the incidence of DVT and PE.
2. Haematoma.
   - Incidence is about 4%.
   - Increases the rate of wound infection.
3. Hip dislocation.
   - Incidence is about 2%.
   - Most dislocations occur within 6 months of surgery.
   - Management is usually conservative, but recurrent dislocation requires revision surgery.
4. Fractures.
   - Overall incidence is about 1%.
   - Include fractures of the femur (when dislocating the hip or inserting the femoral component), acetabulum and pubic rami.
5. Sciatic nerve injury.
   - Incidence is less than 1%.
   - Occurs intra-operatively or post-operatively following dislocation.

Late complications.

1. Infection.
   - Incidence is about 1.5%.
   - Methods of reducing infection rate include:
     i) Prophylactic broad-spectrum antibiotics, e.g. i.v. cefuroxime at induction and two doses post-operatively.
     ii) Gentamicin-impregnated cement.
     iii) Ultra-clean air enclosures – deep infection requires revision surgery.

2. Loosening.
   - Incidence is about 35% at 15-year follow-up.

- Due to absorption of cement around the implant.
- Hypersensitivity, low grade infection and imperfect prosthetic design may be causative factors.
- Loosening usually presents with pain but radiological changes are usually present before presentation.

3. Idiopathic heterotopic bone formation.
   - Incidence is about 10%.
   - Reduces range of movement.
   - Indomethacin given post-operatively may reduce the incidence.

Other complications
These include fracture of the femur during surgery, bed sores, urinary retention and infection, postoperative mental confusion, ectopic periarticular ossification and other respiratory and cardiovascular complications.

---

3. The indications for surgery and surgical treatment of duodenal ulceration

Indications for surgery
1. Failure of medical management.
2. Recurrent ulceration.
3. Development of complications such as perforation, haemorrhage and gastric outflow obstruction.

Surgical options for duodenal ulceration
1. Highly selective vagotomy (HSV). In this procedure the acid secreting parietal cells of the stomach are denervated. Therefore no drainage procedure is required (unless there is associated gastric outflow obstruction due to duodenal scarring).
   - The mortality is less than 0.5%.
   - The recurrence rate is approximately 7%.
   - Diarrhoea and dumping are relatively rare with this procedure.
   - Lesser curve necrosis may complicate 0.2% of cases.

2. Truncal vagotomy and drainage. In this procedure both vagal trunks (anterior and posterior) are divided and pyloroplasty or gastrojejunostomy is carried out.
   - The recurrence rate is approximately 7%.
   - Dumping and/or diarrhoea may affect 25% of cases.

3. Truncal vagotomy and antrectomy.
   - This procedure has the lowest recurrence rate (less than 1%) and is popular in the USA.
   - Dumping occurs in 25% and diarrhoea in 10%.

4. Selective vagotomy and drainage. In this operation the hepatic and coeliac branches of the vagus are preserved. It is not widely used.

5. Posterior vagotomy and seromyotomy of the lesser curve.
   - It has similar results to HSV but easier to perform.

The surgical treatment for complications of duodenal ulceration
1. Perforation is treated with simple closure incorporating an amental patch and combined with peritoneal lavage. A definitive anti-ulcer treatment (truncal vagotomy and pyloroplasty or HSV) is also

performed in patients who perforate whilst on H_2 antagonists.

2. Haemorrhage is treated with pyloroduodonotomy, under-running of the bleeding vessel and ulcer with a non-absorbable suture and a definitive anti-ulcer procedure in the form of HSV, truncal vagotomy and pyloroplasty or Polya gastrectomy.
   - endoscopic treatment with laser, bipolar diathermy, adrenaline or ethanol injection is an alternative.

3. Gastric outflow obstruction is treated with truncal vagotomy combined with pyloroplasty or gastrojejunostomy. Alternatives include HSV with duodonoplasty and Polya gastrectomy.

---

4. Surgical options for ulcerative colitis

Indications for surgery
1. Malignant change.
2. Toxic megacolon.
3. Dysplasia.
4. Fulminating colitis with risk of perforation.
5. Failure of medical management.

Options
1. Proctocolectomy with ileostomy.
   Advantages
   - Diseased tissue is removed.
   - Risk of malignancy is eliminated.

   Disadvantages
   - Permanent stoma.
   - Sexual dysfunction may complicate surgery.
   - Problems with perineal wound healing.

2. Total colectomy with ileorectal anastomosis.
   - Seldom performed nowadays.
   - No permanent stoma.
   - Malignancy may develop in the rectum.

3. Proctocolectomy with continent ileostomy.
   - Ileal reservoir is fashioned with a valve mechanism.
   - High incidence of incontinence.

4. Restorative protocolectomy with ileal reservoir.
   - Colon and rectum are removed to the level of pelvic floor. The remainder of the rectum is removed through transanal mucosectomy. The apex of the ileal reservoir is anastomosed to the anal canal.
   - Suitable for young patients (<60) with intact anal sphincter mechanism. Crohn's disease is a contraindication.
   - Various types of pouches are used, e.g. S, J or W pouch.
   - Antidiarrhoeal drugs are usually required.
   - It is becoming the procedure of choice with improvement in the quality of life.

- Post-operative complications include pelvic sepsis (12%), small bowel obstruction due to adhesions, anastomotic stricture (10%) and pouchitis (10%).

5. Total colectomy with mucous fistula (Stage I) and ileal reservoir (Stage II) in critically ill patients.

---

5. Surgical audit

Definition

- It is the critical and systematic analysis of quality of surgical care; the aim being to improve the standards of surgical care.
- Most audits (in clinical practice) represent retrospective studies.

Types of studies

1. Audit of structure. This refers to the organization and availability of resources to deliver the surgical service.
2. Audit of process. This refers to the way the patient has been received and managed from admission to discharge.
3. Audit of outcome. This refers to the result of surgical intervention.

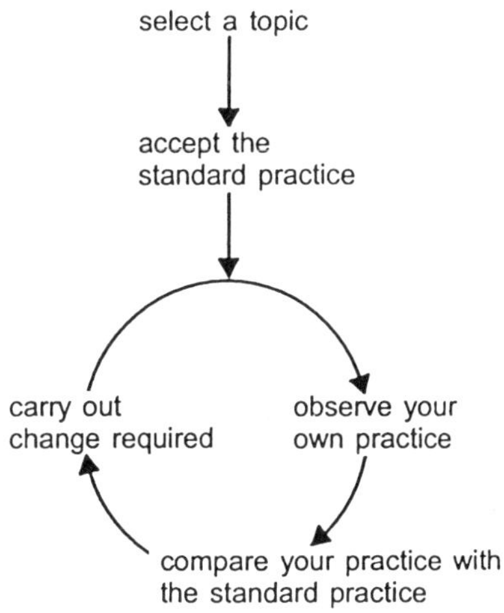
select a topic
accept the
standard practice
observe your
own practice
compare your practice with
the standard practice
carry out
change required

Figure. Audit cycle

Stages of audit

1. Primary data collection.
   - This is best performed by an audit sister.
   - Doctors are less accurate than nursing staff in recording primary data.
   - Audit forms that have a special section for post-operative complications are widely used.

2. Verification of primary data through confidential peer review.

3. Submission of data to analysis.
   - Computers are of great value at this stage.

Audit meetings
- Should be held regularly, e.g. fortnightly.
- Should be attended by all members of the surgical team.
- Inclusion of nursing staff (theatre and surgical wards) is useful, but should not affect confidentiality.

Characteristics of a successful audit
1. Complete.
2. Honest.
3. Accurate.
4. Educational.
5. Confidential.
6. Objective.
7. Reproducible.
8. Cost-effective.

6. Diagnostic peritoneal lavage

Indications

1. Unconscious multiple trauma patients.
2. Unexplained shock in multiple trauma patients.
3. Blunt abdominal injuries with equivocal physical signs.
4. Suspected abdominal injury in intoxicated patients.
5. Other injuries such as spinal cord and thoraco-abdominal injuries.

Contraindications

1. Pregnancy.
2. Previous laparotomy.
3. Morbid obesity.
4. Obvious abdominal injuries necessitating laparotomy.

Method

1. Empty stomach (NG tube) and bladder (catheterization) if necessary.
2. Prepare the abdomen with povidone-iodine and drape with sterile towels.
3. Infiltrate lignocaine and adrenalin in the infraumbilical skin and underlying parietes.
4. Make a 2–3 cm incision in the infraumbilical region in the midline down to the linea alba.
5. Pick up the peritoneum with forceps and insert a purse string. Then make a small incision in the peritoneum and insert a multiperforated polythene tube through it. The tube is directed at 45° into the pelvis.
6. Tighten the purse string and introduce normal saline through the tube (500 ml in children and 1000 ml in adults) with the patient in a slight Trendelenberg position.
7. After 10 minutes, syphon fluid from peritoneal cavity.
8. Positive lavage:
   a) RBC count $>100{,}000/\text{mm}^3$.
   b) Grossly blood-stained fluid.
   c) WCC count $>500/\text{mm}^3$.
   d) Amylase level >200 units.

Notes:

1. Peritoneal lavage is to be preferred to peritoneal tap.
2. False-positive results are rare in peritoneal lavage.
3. Retroperitoneal haemorrhage may produce a false-negative result.

7. The clinical features and treatment of meconium ileus

- Thick sticky meconium becomes impacted in the distal ileum.
- Meconium ileus is the neonatal presentation of cystic fibrosis in approximately 13% of patients.

Clinical features

1. Meconium peritonitis is due to intrauterine perforation.
2. Acute bowel obstruction in the neonate with abdominal distension, bile-stained vomiting and absolute constipation.
3. Abdominal radiographs may show distended loops of small bowel and mottled ground-glass appearance of impacted meconium.
4. Perforation may occur leading to peritonitis.

Treatment

1. Correction of dehydration and nasogastric tube may be required.
2. It may be possible to clear the meconium by installation of Gastrografin per rectum under radiological control.
3. Surgery is indicated if the above treatment fails or if perforation develops. The surgical treatment consists of laparotomy, ileotomy and removal of impacted meconium. If the impacted ileal segment is gangrenous then resection of the ischaemic bowel is required. Peritoneal lavage with normal saline is carried out for peritonitis if present. Temporary ileostomy is occasionally performed.
4. The patient is started on pancreatin postoperatively.

---

8. Hazards of blood transfusion

1. Allergic reaction.
   - Due to anti-IgA antibodies and other antibodies against serum proteins.
   - Vary in severity from urticarial wheals to circulatory shock.
   - Adrenaline may be required.

2. Febrile reactions.
   - Due to antibodies against leukocytes and platelets. The antibodies are directed against HLA-antigens.
   - Usually present with a rise in temperature.
   - Leukocyte-poor blood may be required.

3. Haemolytic reactions.
   - Mostly due to blood incompatibility (e.g. incorrect labelling).
   - Reactions may be immediate or delayed (occurring a few weeks later).
   - In the immediate reactions four phases may be identified: 1) haemolytic shock; 2) post-shock phase (haemoglobinuria/ jaundice); 3) oliguric phase; and 4) diuretic phase.
   - Managed by stopping transfusion, i.v. frusemide, compatible RBC transfusion with plasma expanders and i.v. hydrocortisone.

4. Reactions of contaminated blood.
   - Contamination occurs through improper collection, storage and administration.
   - Endotoxaemic shock may occur.
   - Gram-positive and Gram-negative bacteria may be responsible.

5. Thrombophlebitis.

6. Air embolism.

7. Transmission of disease.
   Examples include hepatitis B (risk reduced with routine screening of blood donations), Ebstein Barr virus, cytomegalovirus (especially in the immunocompromised, e.g. hepatitis), non-A non-B hepatitis, malaria, syphilis, brucellosis, toxoplasmosis and most importantly HIV.

8. Haemosiderosis occurs after repeated transfusions for chronic anaemia.

9. Circulatory overload.
   - Risk patients include the elderly, infants, patients with chronic anaemia, cardiac or respiratory disease.
   - Careful monitoring may prevent the complication.

10. Massive blood transfusion reactions.
    - When the blood transfusion volume over 12 hours equals the volume of patient blood.
    - Blood (ACD) storage at 4°C leads to loss of function of platelets and factor V and VIII. pH and K^+ levels increase.
    - Citrate in the transfused blood reduces the concentration of ionized Ca^{2+} in the platelet plasma.
    - Cardiac dysrhythmia is a recognized complication.
    - Thrombocytopaenia requires platelets transfusion.
    - Disseminated intravascular coagulopathy (DIC) (therefore for every 5–10 units of stored blood transfused, 1 unit of fresh blood should be given, also 10 ml of 10% calcium gluconate is given).